Pegan Diet

Meal Plan For 7 Days To Reduce Inflammation, Balance
Hormones, And Improve Overall Health

*(Quick And Tasty Recipes For Healthy Eating And Feeling
Great)*

Rueben Nicholson

TABLE OF CONTENT

Vegan And Pegan Are Equivalent To The Pegan Diet.

To maximize the health benefits of vegetarian and vegan diets, Pegan places an emphasis on whole, unprocessed ingredients. Boxed goods are incompatible with vegan diets. Dr. Mark Hyman designed them. Many of the foods that you will purchase will not contain any nutritional information. You are more inclined to shop along the perimeter of the supermarket.

Pegan dietary principles emphasize the consumption of locally sourced, organic, and sustainably produced foods. During your Pegan journey, you may discover that you appreciate visiting local farmers' markets or grocery stores with extensive organic produce sections. You will gain a greater appreciation for nutritious foods and be forced to abandon your comfort zone.

The Pegan diet reduces inflammation and maintains a healthy blood sugar level for optimal health. According to proponents of the Pegan lifestyle, it has numerous health benefits, including weight loss, increased energy levels, and the reduction of chronic diseases like diabetes, heart disease, and obesity.

Advantages Of The Vegan Diet

The pegan diet is associated with enhanced health in a few scientifically proven ways, but it has not been clinically proven as a whole. Emphasis on fruits and vegetables as the foundation of the diet is one of its greatest nutritional advantages.

Fruits and vegetables are, without a doubt, among the most nutrient-dense foods, containing a variety of vitamins, minerals, plant compounds, and fiber that may aid in preventing disease and reducing inflammation in the body.

Pegan diets emphasize the consumption of natural fat sources, such as seafood caught in the wild, nuts, seeds, avocados, and olives. These nutrients are good for the heart.

Reducing the consumption of processed foods, which contain a variety of added carbohydrates and preservatives, improves the nutritional quality of the diet while removing potentially harmful additives, pesticides, and chemicals.

Negative Aspects of the Vegan Diet

The vegan diet has been endorsed by Parsley Health for its nutritional benefits. However, some individuals may not benefit from eliminating gluten and dairy.

Even though it is known that a number of these foods promote inflammation, excluding entire food groups may result in nutrient depletion and unnecessary restriction for those who do not have an intolerance.

It may not be necessary to restrict the consumption of legumes and gluten-free cereals, both of which provide distinct health benefits. In order to satisfy the protein and carbohydrate needs of endurance athletes, it may be necessary to include foods that are restricted in the paste diet.

If you have any concerns regarding these specific restrictions, it is always advisable to consult a health coach or physician.

Think Of Sugar As A Recreational Narcotic

A key principle of the Pegan diet is to limit the consumption of added carbohydrates, which are frequently present in processed and refined foods. To treat sugar as a recreational drug while adhering to the Pegan diet, consider the following suggestions.

• Steer clear of processed and packaged foods, as they frequently contain high levels of added carbohydrates. Focus instead on consuming whole, unprocessed foods like fruits, vegetables, nuts, seeds, and whole grains.

• Carefully read food labels and select foods low in added sugars. Avoid goods that contain sugar, corn syrup, honey, or molasses in prominent positions on the ingredient list.

• Experiment with small quantities of natural sweeteners such as stevia, honey, and maple syrup to sweeten foods and beverages. These sweeteners are typically less refined than white sugar and have a lower glycemic index.

• Watch your portion sizes and avoid consuming excessive quantities of sugary foods and beverages. If sugar is treated as a recreational substance, it should be consumed infrequently and in moderation.

• Engage in mindful dining and be aware of your body's sugar response. Consuming sugary foods can induce a "sugar rush" and lead to feelings of jitteriness, anxiety, or irritability. If you observe these effects, consider consuming fewer foods that are healthier.

sugar and choose substitutes

Importantly, the Pegan diet is a flexible and individualized approach to eating, and the specific guidelines for treating sugar as a recreational substance may vary based on your personal preferences and health objectives. If you are uncertain about how to follow the Pegan diet or if you have health concerns, it is always best to consult with a healthcare provider or registered dietitian who can offer personalized advice and support.

ELEVEN

Don't rely on caffeine and alcohol

On the Pegan diet, coffee and alcohol are discouraged because they contain added sugars and other unhealthy elements. To avoid relying on these beverages while following the Pegan diet, consider the following:

• Choose organic, fair trade, and shade-grown coffee and limit your daily consumption to one or two glasses. • Opt for low-sugar, low-alcohol wines and beers, and limit your weekly consumption to one or two beverages. Cocktails and mixed beverages often contain added sugars and other unhealthy ingredients, so they should be avoided.

• Experiment with alternative beverages, such as coconut water and vegetable liquids, to diversify your diet and promote your health.

• Be aware of your body's reaction to stimulants and alcohol, and pay attention to its signals. It is crucial to consume these substances in moderation to avoid negative effects on your health and well-being, as they can influence your mood, energy levels, and sleep.

It is essential to note that the Pegan diet is a personalized dietary plan, with guidelines for and alcohol varying based on your personal preferences and health objectives. If you are uncertain about how to follow the Pegan diet, or if you have any health concerns, it is always a flexible and approach to the specific avoiding coffee best to consult with a healthcare provider or registered dietitian, who can offer personalized advice and support.

Utilize Individualized Nutrition For Optimal Health

Individual dietary requirements, preferences, and objectives are taken into account by personalized nutrition. To achieve optimal health through personalized nutrition on the Pegan diet, consider the following strategies:

• Consult with a healthcare provider or registered dietitian who can assist you in comprehending your nutritional needs and developing a plan that is tailored to your specific objectives and health concerns.

• Be aware of your body's response to various foods and beverages, and pay attention to your body's signals. Consider how you feel after consuming and drinking, and avoid foods and beverages that make you feel ill or uneasy.

• Experiment with various varieties of foods and beverages and record what works and what doesn't. Don't be afraid to attempt new foods and recipes, and be willing to make dietary adjustments based on your body's reaction.

• Consider your age, gender, level of activity, and medical conditions when devising your individualized nutrition plan. These factors can affect your nutritional demands and may necessitate dietary modifications.

• Focus on consuming a variety of whole, unprocessed foods and avoid refined and processed foods that are high in added sugars, sodium, and unhealthy lipids.

It is essential to note that the Pegan diet is a flexible and individualized approach to eating, and that the specific guidelines for utilizing personalized nutrition may vary depending on your personal preferences and health objectives. If you are uncertain about how to follow the Pegan diet, or if you have health concerns, it is always best to consult with a healthcare provider or registered dietician who can offer personalized advice and support.

SECTION THIRTEEN

How to Detox, Cleanse, and Reset Wisely?

Cleansing, detoxifying, and resetting can be beneficial for promoting overall health and well-being, but it is essential to do so carefully to avoid negative health effects. To detoxify, detox, and reset intelligently while on the Pegan diet, consider the following suggestions:

Before beginning a detoxification, detox, or reset program, consult a healthcare professional or registered dietitian. These programs can be restrictive and may not be suitable for all individuals, depending on their health and nutritional requirements.

• Select a program that is risk-free, well-rounded, and supported by scientific evidence. Diets that promise fast fixes or rapid weight loss can be harmful to your health, so avoid them.

• Prioritize consuming a variety of whole, unprocessed foods, including fruits, vegetables, nuts, seeds, and whole grains. These nutrient-dense foods can support the body's natural detoxification processes.

• Steer clear of processed and refined foods as well as those high in added sugars, sodium, and unhealthy lipids. These foods can be detrimental to your health and can negate the effects of a cleansing, detox, or reset program.

• Observe your body's response to the program and pay attention to its signals. If you experience any adverse effects, such as vertigo, fatigue, or digestive issues, discontinue the program and consult a physician or registered dietitian.

It is essential to remember that the Pegan diet is a flexible and individualized eating plan, and the specific guidelines for purifying, detoxing, and resetting can vary depending on your personal preferences and health objectives. If you are uncertain about how to follow the Pegan diet or if you have health concerns, it is always best to consult with a healthcare provider or registered dietitian who can offer personalized advice and support.

PARAGRAPHA FOURTEEN

Evaluate the risks and benefits of a vegan diet.

A vegan diet excludes all animal products, including meat, poultry, seafood, eggs, and dairy. To evaluate the hazards and benefits of a vegan diet, you can take into account the following elements:

• Nutritional sufficiency: A well-planned vegan diet can provide the body with all the nutrients necessary for optimal health. However, it is essential to consume enough protein, vitamins B12 and D, calcium, and iron, as well as other nutrients typically found in animal products.

A vegan diet can be more sustainable and environmentally beneficial than a diet containing animal products. Vegan diets require less water, land, and energy to produce, and can reduce emissions of greenhouse gases and other environmental contaminants.

• Ethical considerations: Many individuals choose a vegan diet because it prevents animal suffering and promotes the humane treatment of animals.

• Personal preferences: A vegan diet may not be suitable for everyone; when deciding whether to follow a vegan diet, it is essential to consider your individual preferences, needs, and goals.

It is essential to note that the risks and benefits of a vegan diet can vary depending on your individual circumstances and how well you plan and implement the diet. Consultation with a healthcare provider or registered dietitian who can provide individualized guidance and support on how to follow a vegan diet safely and effectively is always recommended.

What Foods Should You Avoid?

The majority of clinical experts would agree that diet is the primary cause of infection. In addition to the immediate consequences such as cardiovascular disease and weight problems, consuming the incorrect food sources causes a variety of other fundamental problems. In the last four decades, the cost of being overweight has increased from 5% to 40%, according to the available data.

In addition, experts have noted that every six out of ten Americans have a tenacious infection, ranging from cancer, heart disease, and clinical depression to Alzheimer's disease and dementia.

Diabetes mellitus, according to clinical experts, is an additional type of persistent illness that has a significant impact on individuals worldwide. There are two types of diabetic issues: one is part of a group of conditions known as 'immune system disease'; this is an incurable condition.

Although the first type is quite common, you should be most concerned about the second. The second type of diabetes is not an immune system disorder - individuals consume so much sugar that their bodies cannot keep up. Currently, the vast majority of the population has Type-2 diabetes or is regarded as pre-diabetic. All of these problems have an impact on the country's intelligence and politics. For example, a large number of Americans manage Type-2 diabetes, and close to 33 percent of Medicare funds are allocated to diabetic issues.

This is a substantial amount of assessment funds allocated to an essential food-related illness.

Approximately seven out of ten applicants for the role of perpetrator are denied because they suffer from diseases like obesity. Numerous children in the United States grow up consuming overly-processed and sugary foods, which causes them to become overweight and experience serious health problems. This is the reason for their discharge from the military.

The cutting-edge food framework has a global impact. A significant portion of our diet consists of unappetizing, uninteresting food varieties.

In the case of prebiotic diet varieties, assuming that you have microscopic intestinal

bacterial excess, clinical experts urge the gradual introduction of these dietary varieties. While the conventional immune system provides a one-size-fits-all solution, the adaptable immune system will definitely provide antigen-specific inputs. A paleo diet can also aid in immune system development by reducing the incidence of antigenic illnesses such as influenza and colds.

The current dietary framework influences the global community. There are a great deal of unappetizing food sources that are hideously processed, and they also make up the majority of our diet.

Milk

When discussing a pegan diet plan, it is suggested that we consider two distinct diet routines: one that adheres to the paleo diet routine and the other that adheres to the vegetarian diet routine. Regarding a vegetarian diet, dairy products are not permitted. This is the reason why milk products are inadequate for the publishing of healthy vegan diet routine components.

Nonetheless, many are confused as to why we should stop drinking milk. It builds strong and healthy bones If milk is not considered healthy and balanced, why is it promoted as such? According to driving-trained professionals, there is no logical basis for it. Indeed, the claimed benefits have also proven to be false. There are real and dangerous risks, such as processing difficulties, dermatitis, hormonal specialist issues, immune system disease, allergies, and malignant growth cells. Myth: Beneficial for the bones.

As children, we were all taught that milk products are the finest sources of calcium, which will provide us with strong, healthy bones and reduce the likelihood of fractures. Clinical experts concur that variation exists. It was discovered that countries with the highest milk consumption, such as Sweden, also had the highest crack prices, while countries with the lowest milk consumption, such as Indonesia and China, had the lowest crack prices. Adults who consumed a daily glass of milk were 9 percent more likely to suffer a fracture, according to additional research.

If you abstain from milk, you may consider alternative sources of calcium and Vitamin D. Initially, milk is fortified with Vitamin D, which is not typically present in the diet. Sunlight, herring, and porcini mushrooms are the most effective sources of vitamin D. On the other hand, you can additionally acquire

Calcium can be obtained from preserved salmon, chia seeds, sardines, sesame seeds, tofu, and unique greens including arugula, collards, and kale.

What dairy products can you consume?

There are very few milk products that can be consumed on occasion. You can try milk products from sheep and goats (or a lucky cow), which contain A2 casein protein that is more flexible and less flammable. However, milk products from cows contain high levels of A1 casein, which can cause dermatitis, skin inflammation, allergic reactions, and growth. In the interim, A2 casein contains glutathione, a potent normal detoxifying, cancer-preventative, and mitigating substance. Whether or not you enjoy cow dairy, it is recommended that you choose grass-fed, regeneratively reared, and full-fat cow products.

Coffee as well as Alcohol

Excessive alcohol and coffee consumption can alter a person's mood, sleep cycle, and chemical balance. Water is the primary beverage your body requires.

The majority of the human body is composed of water; if you do not consume enough water, it can lead to a variety of diseases. Regardless of whether you need to add flavor to your water, you can add cucumber or citrus, or prepare chilled natural teas. While a vegan diet allows you to consume alcohol-infused water, the best beverage to consume is plain water.

In contrast, you can also dissolve electrolytes in water; electrolytes are types of minerals that allow you to replenish your mass and nerves, thereby assisting with waste elimination, cell reproduction, pH balance, and hydration. Remember electrolytes for water after exercise to rehydrate your body and replenish the minerals you lost during exercise.

Coffee

Coffee is considered one of the finest sources of cell reinforcements, which can be used to determine the decreased level of anti-oxidants in our diets. Studies have shown that coffee can reduce the likelihood of a variety of health conditions, including Parkinson's disease, dementia, and cardiovascular disease.

However, coffee does not benefit everyone. Generally speaking, coffee can increase insulin production, particularly in individuals with Type 2 diabetes. It can also contribute to hormonal damage by increasing stress hormones such as cortisol.

If you experience heart palpitations, agitation, or other types of energy issues, it may be time to examine your coffee consumption. It is advisable to abstain from alcohol consumption periodically throughout the year. Many of us have become so dependent on irrefutable levels of caffeine that we cannot start the day without a cup of coffee. It has been demonstrated that a normal day can be experienced without the beverage.

As an alternative to espresso, you can experiment with a variety of other types of beverages. Tea is an excellent option because it contains powerful phenolic compounds that protect our cardiovascular system and combat disease. Similarly, if you cannot exist without coffee, consume it without flavorings and sugars. Alcohol

As red wine contains resveratrol, it is considered by many to be the superior alternative to intoxicant. This substance can also be found in a variety of dietary supplements and edibles.

It has been studied that alcohol has a much greater impact on women than on men; research has confirmed that women who consume a lot of alcohol are significantly more likely to develop breast cancer. In addition, it impairs the existing nutrients in your body as well as your mind, stomach, and liver. In contrast to normal conviction, alcohol does not help you fall asleep; in fact, it may take you longer to fall asleep, and your pulse rate remains elevated throughout the night.

Consequently, you should eliminate alcoholic beverages. , if you are unable to do so, treat liquor as you would sugar; an occasional glass is acceptable. Burning through every day will unquestionably become dangerous. If you don't feel great after consuming alcohol, you must stop immediately. There is no pity in letting people know that you do not consume alcohol or that you have ceased. Even if there is peer pressure, find a way to say no and let them know you're already having a good time without consuming alcohol.

Blanc Flour

When we discuss sugar in this section, we do not mean beetroot sugar; rather, we refer to walking natural sweetener. However, unlike beet sugar and high-fructose corn syrup, unprocessed sweetener is not genetically modified.

However, both are believed to have similar effects on increasing the body's insulin levels, which can lead to weight gain (belly fat), fatty liver, and pre-diabetic complications such as insulin obstruction, diabetes, high cholesterol, etc.

There is no disinfectant in white sugar; however, white flour is blanched. The carbohydrates in sugar walking stick are managed by removing the nutrients and minerals, which are referred to as molasses; the remaining substance is essentially white sugar. If you don't have them, your body will definitely use them from its reserves to neutralize the sugar.

Similarly, when flour is enhanced, minerals and nutrients are extracted from the body. As a result of the fact that numerous flours are fortified, they will contain some synthetic nutrients and iron; however, this is not the type of iron the body requires. These supplements can impede the body, especially if you are allergic to iron.

It is a remarkable feat for the body to eliminate iron, as it tends to accumulate instead of being eliminated. Consequently, if you are consuming foods with excess iron in the wrong asset, the trend can result in a variety of potential issues. Similar to whole wheat flour, white flour utilizes batter conditioners to make batter extremely easy to convert into breads and pastries. Alloxan is a compound that kills the cells in the pancreas that make insulin, causing Type-1 diabetes in rodents like hamsters and mice. Benzoyl peroxide is additionally utilized as a part of the flour.

Additionally, flour contains the hazardous substance potassium bromate, which is banned in Europe, Brazil, China, and Canada. According to research, potassium bromate causes malignant growth cells in animals. When making breads, croissants, or cookies, the synthetic is added to white flour to create the ideal surface of the dough. Lastly, white flour also contains gluten; a large number of people on the planet today have a sensitivity to gluten. Gluten can activate immune system disorders and aggravate the digestive tract.

When white is contrasted with black, the most recent case exhibits a greater number of problems than the prior case.

Sugar and refined white flour.

Getting Rid Of Sugar Cravings

Many individuals struggle to eliminate sugar cravings ordinarily. Due to their sugar cravings, a small number of individuals are unable to adhere to diet plans.

There will come a time when your craving for sugar, especially for carbohydrates such as sweets, cereals, bread, and pasta, will be overwhelming. If you want to eliminate your sugar cravings, there are four key steps you can take. This consists of:

1. Diet strategy.

Everything begins with your daily dietary regimen. Adding foods to your diet that can regulate your blood glucose levels in a manner similar to insulin is the underlying principle you should pursue. Currently, insulin is a chemical that functions in the body alongside the pancreas. to reduce glucose levels. The primary problem faced by diabetics is that they cannot consume or that their insulin receptor sites are not functioning properly; it is also conceivable that their body is not producing enough insulin.

If you want to surmount your sugar cravings, you must control your insulin levels and maintain constant glucose levels. To accomplish this, you need to add three items to your diet: healthy and balanced fat, solid protein, and fiber. These three supplements will aid in preventing an increase in glucose levels and reducing sugar cravings. Additionally, you will definitely feel complete longer.

Natural, grass-fed hamburger, wild poultry and chicken, and free-range eggs are exceptional sources of protein. You may also select aged dairy products. These dietary sources will help you obtain natural and high-quality solid proteins. Increasing one's protein intake will effectively reduce sugar desires.

Next, you need to consume healthy, balanced lipids. Nuts and seeds are viable options; flax seeds and chia seeds that have been developed are particularly intriguing. Other wonderful sources of healthy and balanced lipids include clarified butter (ghee), avocados, coconut oil, and almonds. Healthy lipids are essential for controlling glucose levels.

Fiber is also essential for controlling blood glucose levels. The many

Successful sources of fiber include seeds, berries, vegetables, and almonds.

2. Getting clear of both sugar and grains from your diet. If you want to decrease your sugar cravings, you should eliminate carbohydrates and grains from your diet. This is a vicious cycle; the more sugar you consume, the more your body requires. When giving up sugar, the initial few days will be the most difficult to endure.

Experts advise that you gradually eliminate sugar from your diet and seek for healthy alternatives to help satisfy your sweet tooth. You can add natural stevia powder or leaves to your diet; these ingredients will help you control your sugar tooth.

Additionally, you can opt for flavored protein powder. Eventually, you must eliminate sugar, grains, and carbohydrates from your body. 3. Using the finest supplements to regulate blood sugar levels. Chromium is an outstanding dietary supplement for diabetic patients. However, consuming 200 micrograms of chromium three times per day can help stabilize blood sugar levels. You can visit online stores and search for high-quality chromium supplements to neutralize your blood glucose levels and reduce your sugar cravings; these supplements can be taken with meals.

Vitamin B is also an option. Taking B-complex vitamins can help curb sugar cravings, particularly Vitamins B6 and B12. Additionally, there are probiotic supplements. These supplements can help reduce sugar cravings because they eliminate yeast from the body. Poor microorganisms and yeast subsist on sugar. The supplement will aid in maintaining yeast homeostasis within the body.

These three types of supplements effectively reduce sugar cravings.

4. Perform the best forms of exercises.

Numerous cardiovascular exercises will increase your desire for sweets. On the other hand, doing isometric or weight-training exercises such as Pilates, yoga, etc. can help maintain blood sugar levels and also do not induce a craving for carbohydrates. You should avoid long-distance cardio exercises, such as running, as they can induce a craving for sugar.

Tips For The Vegan Diet When Eating Out

The Pegan diet promotes the ingestion of plant-based proteins such as legumes, beans, nuts, and seeds. Look for these plant-based proteins, such as a vegetarian burger or a black bean burrito, when dining out.

Avoid Refined cereals The Pegan diet prohibits refined cereals such as white flour and white rice. Instead, choose whole cereals such as quinoa and brown rice.

3. Load Up on Veggies: When following the Pegan diet, vegetables should always be the main course. Choose vegetable-rich dishes, such as salads and stir-fries.

4. Avoid Added Sugars: Added sugars are not part of the Pegan diet, so avoid specialty coffees, beverages, and desserts that contain added sugars.

Ask Questions: Do not be afraid to inquire about the food's preparation. Inquire if there are any added sugars, oils, or other ingredients that may not be suitable for a vegan diet.

The Pegan diet encourages the consumption of healthful fats such as avocados, olive oil, and nuts. Be sure to order dishes that contain these healthful fats when dining out.

Consequently, it is possible to dine out while adhering to a vegan diet. By adhering to these guidelines, you can ensure that your diet is both nutritious and delectable.

This page purposely lacked content

Recipes for Pegan Diet Days 1-7: The Pegan Diet Transition
Day 1: Inform Yourself

Educating yourself about what the Pegan Diet entails and what it entails is the first step in making the switch. Read about the Pegan Diet and become familiar with its guidelines and principles. Discover which foods are included and excluded, the diet's benefits, and how to make the switch.

Day 2: Create a Shopping List

Create a grocery list of the foods you need to stock your pantry and refrigerator based on the meals you will be consuming. This will help you remain on track and ensure you have all the necessary ingredients and supplies to transition to the Pegan Diet.

Day Three: Empty Your Pantry

Remove from your pantry and refrigerator all foods that are incompatible with the Pegan Diet. This includes all processed foods, refined sugars, white flour, and foods with added sugars, artificial sweeteners, or unhealthy lipids.

Day Four: Stock Up on Nutritious Foods

Go grocery shopping and stock up on all the healthful Pegan Diet-compliant foods. This includes fruits, vegetables, whole cereals, nuts and seeds, and plant-based proteins.

Start meal planning on Day 5

Start planning your weekly menus now. Include breakfast, lunch, and supper, as well as snacks. Plan scrumptious and nutrient-dense meals that adhere to the Pegan Diet's guidelines.

Day 6: Commence cooking

Commence preparing dishes for the week. Include an abundance of whole foods in your diet and avoid processed and refined foods. Utilize healthy lipids, such as olive oil and coconut oil, and prioritize high-fiber, nutrient-rich foods.

Day 7: Festivities

You have successfully completed the first week of the Pegan Diet transition! Commemorate this achievement and reflect on your progress. Consider how consuming clean, whole foods for one week has affected your energy levels and disposition.

Congratulations on taking the initial step toward adopting a vegan diet!

Introducing New Foods and Experimenting with Recipes, Days 8-14 Day 8 marks the beginning of incorporating novel foods into your diet. Start by selecting one novel food to sample. Verify that there are no allergens or ingredients you dislike by reading the ingredient list thoroughly. Then, prepare the cuisine per the instructions. Determine if you enjoy the cuisine by sampling it.

Choose another novel food to try on Day 9. Read the ingredient list carefully and compare it to the food you ate the day before. Again, prepare the food according to the instructions. Enjoy!

Try out a new recipe on Day 10. Choose a dish that incorporates some of the new foods you've recently sampled. Be sure to peruse the instructions thoroughly and adhere to them precisely. Consider the cuisine according to your tastes.

Try an alternate recipe on day 11. Choose a dish that incorporates some of the new foods you've recently sampled. Again, carefully read the instructions and obey them. Determine if you like the dish by trying it out.

Choose a new recipe for Day 12 that includes some of the same ingredients you've been using. Compare the instructions to previous preparations you have attempted. Prepare the dish and observe how it tastes.

Choose a new recipe for Day 13 that includes some of the same ingredients you've been using. Read and follow the instructions attentively. Determine if you like the dish by trying it out.

Day 14: Use some of the same ingredients you've been using in a new recipe. Compare the instructions to previous preparations you have attempted. Prepare the dish and observe how it tastes. You have now attempted four new recipes and are becoming accustomed to cooking with new ingredients. Congratulations!

You will have attempted at least eight new foods and four new recipes by the end of the two weeks. In addition, you will have gained confidence in your ability to cook with new ingredients and experiment with various recipes. Well done!

1.6 Benefit

The Pegan diet emphasizes the consumption of healthy, natural ingredients. It aims to avoid refined foods and most animal-based products in favor of consuming more fruits and vegetables. Because there are no clear and fast rules regarding what is and is not acceptable, the focus is on making excellent lifestyle decisions. The Pegan diet also excludes gluten, an important source of antioxidants, fiber, vitamins, and minerals.

And it's not just the food; the Pegan diet is loaded with supplements and powders that are meant to replace meals. Although many of us are nutritionally deficient, the best way to obtain nutrients is through food.

There is no doubt that vegans and vegetarians can consume a wide variety of fruits and vegetables, but it may be difficult to reach their daily protein requirements. This diet is lacking in numerous essential nutrients, including manganese, zinc, and vitamin B6.

Benefits Of Pegan Diet

Using Manipulation to Improve Health –

You may consume packaged and processed foods if you wish, but you should generally avoid them. By eliminating processed foods from one's diet, one's body will become more in tune with its natural equilibrium and be able to recover from any health issues.

Focusing on natural foods and avoiding food additives and preservatives can prevent diabetes, cardiovascular disease, high blood pressure, chronic pain, and dementia. You can reduce your risk of these diseases and slow down the aging process by focusing on natural, nutritious foods.

Weight loss - The Pegan diet permits weight loss by prohibiting highly processed and processed foods. It is one of its primary goals, and it enables a healthful approach to weight loss that requires minimal effort. To lose weight healthily, the emphasis is on making healthy decisions.

The Pegan diet emphasizes natural foods and incorporates a variety of healthful seasonings. It encourages the use of more spices in dishes and recipes, which is heart-healthy. Cinnamon, cloves, cumin, nutmeg, and black pepper have been shown to reduce LDL cholesterol and triglyceride levels in the blood.

Cancer prevention - The Pegan diet contains an abundance of nutrients that promote health. It encourages you to consume more vegetables, grains, and fruits, as well as seasonings. Among other spices, cinnamon, cloves, cumin, nutmeg, and black pepper have lower LDL cholesterol and triglyceride levels in the blood. Cinnamon, cloves, cumin, and black pepper have been found to prevent cancer by inhibiting cancer cell proliferation. Enhancing cognitive function - The Pegan diet improves health by assisting your body in making the most efficient use of energy. It encourages you to consume more spices, which is advantageous for your brain's performance. It has been demonstrated that spices such as those listed above aid in memory and learning.

1.7 10 Tips for Sustainable Food Consumption on a Budget

Produce your own

It requires little effort and no nursery to grow a few pots of your beloved herbs and vegetables, which is extremely satisfying. You can grow on various surfaces, including windowsills, patios, and carports. Start with spices, which may be costly but take up little space.

Consider reusing your empty egg cartons as seedling growers and old bean jars and milk bottles as plant containers. A single container of fresh herbs may last up to three months and costs approximately $10. Thyme, rosemary, parsley, and basil are among the herbs contained in the large pots, which emit a variety of fragrances.

They are simple to cultivate; simply maintain them in a bright location year-round, water them frequently, and prune the leaves as necessary. You can now garnish your dishes with fresh herbs for a small fee.

Consume less meat

When it comes to purchasing natural products, flesh ranks first. Natural certification from the Soil Association guarantees that the meat is natural and heavily subsidized by the government. Because meat is costly, but less of it, concentrate on vegetables. When purchasing meat, choose the less expensive cuts, such as shoulder and stomach, which take longer to prepare but are often more flavorful. One of the most effective methods to conserve organic food is to consume less meat.

Meat is high in saturated fat, which contributes to cardiovascular disease and malignancy. It is one of the simplest ways to consume organic foods and reduce your carbon footprint. Meat is a dietary source with a high carbon footprint, so consuming less of it will reduce your food miles.

It is prudent to purchase free-range livestock and even organic poultry. What one pays for is always what one receives. If you purchase the least expensive meat, you are paying for the feed it consumed, which was most likely junk food.

decrease waste

Due to stumbling around the larder, overbuying, and hopeless hoarding, the average household wastes 20-30% of their food. It is a strategy for procuring natural, higher-quality food on a budget. Start your meal plan with your best-seasoned meat and vegetables and build around them. You are drawn to the oldest vegetables in your refrigerator and add fruit to them prior to preparing.

Buy in quantity

Buying in quantity as opposed to one item at a time enables one to acquire more. It is more beneficial and economical for you. If you have less money, you can buy more food in abundance. If necessary, you can always store the remaining vegetables and fruits in a cool, dry location. You can help the environment by reducing food waste, as many vendors lack a clean, cold place to store excess vegetables and fruits. It will benefit both yourself and the environment.

Buy in season

As you may know, seasonal ingredients are the foundation of all the best recipe ideas. If you're like the rest of us, you know what to cook but are unaware of which fruits and vegetables are in season. You will go grocery shopping without considering whether the squash or pears will last long enough to be consumed. Some applications will tell you what fruits and vegetables are in season and where you can obtain the freshest produce in your current location. Frozen fruits and vegetables should be purchased.

If you're on a tight budget, frozen fruits and vegetables, especially out-of-season items such as berries in the winter, are a fantastic option because they are less costly than fresh food. Waiting until the fruit goes on discount is probably too late.

Prepare food from start

If you take care of the condiments and use them sparingly, comfort food varieties are more expensive than cooking from fresh. You prefer to prepare excess portions of meals for lunch the following day or to freeze for later consumption.

Recognize the 'Clean fifteen.'

The Environmental Working Group has released a list known as the 'clean fifteen,' which identifies the vegetables with the least pesticide residue. Avocados, sweet corn, pineapples, cabbage, frozen peas, onions, asparagus, mangoes, papayas, kiwis, eggplant, melon, citrus, cauliflower, and yams are the best non-natural fruits and vegetables to buy if you can't stomach purchasing all-natural items.

The foods that should be avoided are apples, strawberries, grapes, celery, peaches, spinach, sweet chile peppers, imported nectarines, cucumbers, cherry tomatoes, imported snap peas, and potatoes.

Join a nearby organic box program.

Neighborhood box programs are not always the most cost-effective option; rather, they must compete with the costs of organic produce at grocery stores. They will provide a solid foundation for the week's meals, save you time purchasing, and support local ranchers. If given the option, choose a carton of vegetables without potatoes. It will provide you with a wider variety of solutions. The imported natural product is significantly more expensive, so avoid shipments that contain imported items. Whenever possible, local foods are grown using organic methods. Because chemicals are not transported very far, the likelihood that they will be applied to soil or sprayed on vegetation is lower than for other substances.

On the other hand, organic foods are rarely found in close proximity or on an island, so you will need to search for them. Local food is more expensive, but of superior quality. Purchasing food from local farms is beneficial to the local economy because it encourages individuals to spend their money locally rather than sending it elsewhere.

Establish an organic purchasing organization or co-op.

Form a group of individuals interested in purchasing organic vegetables and establish a center. Your purchasing power will increase because you will have more money to spend. It will also allow you to purchase from co-utilizable wholesalers like Essential-exchange and Suma center. Communities are an effective business and cooperation paradigm that may also help you save money as an individual.

If purchasing organic is not an option, ensure that the food is pesticide-free by washing it prior to consumption.

prudent shoppers should avoid supermarkets

Natural food is viewed as beneficial, but it may be prohibitively expensive. Due to the peril posed by convenience stores, it is best to avoid them. Write down the prices of the items you frequently purchase and compare them to the prices of online natural products stores, farmers markets, and greengrocers to determine who offers the most affordable foodstuffs.

Chia Seed Pudding With A Combination Of Berries And Almonds

This creamy and satisfying breakfast pudding is prepared with chia seeds, which are an excellent source of fiber and omega-3 fatty acids. It is topped with a colorful and flavorful berry mixture and crunchy nuts.

Preparation requires five minutes

The setting of chia seed pudding requires refrigeration.

Ingredients:

1/4 cup chia seeds

1 cup of desired milk (such as almond or coconut milk).

1 teaspoon honey or syrup

0.5 ounces of assorted berries (including strawberries, raspberries, and blueberries).

1/4 cup nut crumbs (such as almonds or walnuts).

In a medium basin, combine the chia seeds, milk, and honey or maple syrup with a whisk.

Cover and refrigerate for at least 2 hours or overnight, or until the chia seeds have expanded and the mixture has become pudding-like.

Before serving, garnish the pudding with the mixed berries and chopped almonds.

What is a vegetarian diet?

The pegan diet is based on the belief that nutrient-dense, whole foods are capable of reducing inflammation, maintaining a healthy blood sugar level, and promoting optimal health.

Like many, you may have concluded that adhering to the paleo and vegan diets simultaneously is impossible; according to this expert, this is a reasonable assumption.

You may have read or heard about the personal experiences of individuals on the Pegan Diet.How intriguing was it?Rather, did you find these tales a little strange?

Additionally, I have a contribution from the "good old days," as some people used to say. I transitioned from a strict vegan diet to a vegetarian diet.

But eventually I yearned for novelty once more, so I decided to adopt the Pegan Diet. Prior to that time, a low-carb and protein-rich diet was acceptable for me. Hence, I must admit that it was initially quite perplexing for me.

Yes, I actually began with a trial-and-error approach because I wasn't positive of the actual outcome, but I hoped something would develop. Did I mention that I attempted it for three weeks? Yes, I did, and then I noticed the desired transformations.

The Pegan Diet is a special diet with a unique set of rules that is less restrictive than the paleo and vegan diets.

It places greater emphasis on eating vegetables and fruit and a moderate quantity of meat, fish, seeds, and nuts, with some legumes included.

As a matter of principle, oils, sugars, and grains that have been heavily processed are prohibited, although a very small quantity may not pose a problem.

The pegan diet is not intended to be followed for a brief period of time. Instead, it strives to be more sustainable so that you can continue to follow it forever.

What does this indicate?

The pegan diet, while based on the principles of the paleo and vegan diets, has its own special guidelines designed to encourage long-term sustainability.

75% of a pegan diet should consist of fruits and vegetables, with the remaining 25% comprised primarily of eggs, meats, healthy fats, such as nuts and seeds, and certain legumes and gluten-free whole grains that can be consumed in limited proportions.

Responsible protein supplier

While this diet principle encourages the consumption of more plant-based foods, adequate animal protein consumption is recommended. Notably, as 75% of diets consist of vegetables and fruits, you are likely to consume less meat than on a typical paleo diet, but more than on a vegan diet.

This diet prohibits the consumption of conventionally produced meats and eggs; instead, it emphasizes grass-fed, pasture-raised beef, poultry, and swine, as well as whole eggs.

 Fish with low mercury levels, such as wild salmon and sardines, are promoted as a superior source of protein.

INTRODUCTION

If you're hosting a vegetarian for dinner, you'll need to double-check your menu to ensure it adheres to two fundamental principles. Food sources derived from flora are acceptable, but food sources derived from animals, such as eggs, cheddar, milk, and nectar, are inaccessible.

Approximately 3% of Americans adhere to a vegetarian diet. Their reasons for consuming in this manner vary. A few vegetarians do so to enhance their health. A plant-based diet may reduce the risk of developing certain diseases. Others avoid meat because they do not want to harm animals or because they are concerned about the environment.

If you've considered adopting a vegetarian diet, you should consider whether this way of eating is appropriate for you. Despite the fact that there are genuine benefits to a vegetarian diet, there are also some disadvantages.

What You Can Consume

On a vegetarian diet, you may consume the following plant-based foods:

Land-based foods Vegetables such as peas, legumes, and lentils

Seeds and nuts

Crops, rice, and noodles

Alternative milks include soymilk, coconut milk, and almond milk.

Vegetable oils

What You Can't Consume

Vegetarians cannot consume any animal-derived culinary products, including:

Hamburger, pork, lamb, and other forms of red meat

Chicken, duck, and various other fowl

Crabs, mollusks, and mussels are fish or crustaceans.

Eggs

Cheddar, margarine

Milk, cream, chilled yogurt, and additional dairy products

Mayonnaise (because it contains egg yolks)

Nectar

Medical Advantages

According to studies, vegetarians have better heart health and a reduced risk of contracting certain infections. Those who abstain from meat have a reduced risk of becoming obese or developing coronary disease, high cholesterol, and hypertension. Vegetarians are also less likely to develop diabetes and certain types of cancer, particularly gastrointestinal tract tumors and breast, ovarian, and uterine cancers in women.

Vegetarianism may help you live longer, especially if you reduce your daily caloric intake as well.

Better weight management may be one explanation for these medical benefits. Vegetarians have a lower body mass index (BMI) than those who consume animal products.

Excellent nutrition is another advantage. Organic foods, vegetables, whole cereals, and nuts are the staples of the diet of a vegetarian. These dietary varieties are rich in fiber, cell reinforcements, and compounds that protect against diseases such as diabetes and cancer.

Dangers

A vegetarian diet is generally healthy, but avoiding animal protein can leave you deficient in certain nutrients, such as protein, calcium, omega-3 unsaturated lipids, zinc, and vitamin B12. Protein is required to regulate all chemical responses in the body. Calcium strengthens bones and teeth. Omega-3 unsaturated lipids maintain healthy cells and protect the heart by preventing coronary disease and stroke. These supplements are especially important for the developing bodies of children and expectant women.

You can find alternatives to the majority of these essential nutrients in plant-based foods such as:

Protein: nuts, soy, legumes, quinoa

Calcium: soy milk, freshly squeezed orange, calcium-fortified tofu, broccoli, kale, almonds

Omega-3 unsaturated fats: flaxseeds, vegetable oils, plant-based enhancements

Iron: tofu, soy seeds, spinach, sustained grains

The body uses nutrient B12, which is challenging to obtain from plant sources alone, to produce red platelets and DNA. B12 is only discovered in creature-related objects. If you are a vegetarian, you may require a supplement to make up for the nutrients you are missing from your diet.

Keep in mind that a vegetarian diet is only as healthy as you make it. Items such as "veggie lover" frozen yogurt, treats, and candies are tempting, but you do not wish to exaggerate. In the event that you consume high-fat and processed food sources and supersize your portions, you will gain weight and may experience a similar number of health issues as those who consume a meat-based diet.

The Most Efficient Way To Become Vegetarian

Are you intrigued by the prospect of a vegetarian diet but unsure of where to begin? You may immediately remove all poultry, meat, eggs, and dairy products if you so choose. Alternately, adopt a more progressive strategy and increase the amount of locally grown foods you consume at each meal.

If the idea of eliminating all animal products from your diet seems overwhelming, try a less stringent approach. Some diets emphasize plant-based foods, but leave room for other sources of nourishment:

Pescatarians abstain from eating meat and poultry, but they do consume fish.

Lacto-ovo vegetarian: plant-based diet that also includes dairy and eggs

Flexitarian: a plant-based diet that occasionally includes animal products.

Your primary care physician or a dietitian can assist you in selecting the appropriate food sources as you begin a vegetarian diet. If you have a long-term condition or if you're pregnant, it's essential to seek the assistance of a specialist in order to ensure that your new diet contains the correct combination of nutrients.

A Brief Introduction To The Paleo And Vegan Diets

If you have prior knowledge of the Paleo and Vegan diets, you may be better able to comprehend the Pegan diet in its entirety.

Dietary advocates of the Paleo diet recommend consuming an abundance of fresh fruits and vegetables, seeds and nuts, lean meats, seafood, and healthy lipids on a daily basis. You should avoid processed foods, sugar, dairy, legumes, cereals, and alcohol.

If you think about it, our progenitors subsisted on whatever the natural world provided. This regimen suggests that you follow the same steps. You may already be aware that vegetables and fruits are rich in minerals, vitamins, antioxidants, and phytonutrients. They ensure that you are adequately protected from life-threatening diseases such as diabetes, cancer, and neurodegeneration, among others. They refer to Omega-3 and monounsaturated lipids as healthy fats. All types of seeds and almonds, fish oil, olive oil, avocados, and grass-fed meat are able to provide the recommended daily allowance. You will avoid obesity and diseases associated with obesity, as well as cognitive impairment. Find some quality protein sources, and your diet will be comprehensive. Grass-fed animals, as well as seafood and poultry, produce lean flesh. flesh obtained from grain-fed animals is more prevalent than flesh from wild animals in modern times. For the development of robust bones and muscles, as well as the enhancement of the immune system, it is essential that the body receive lean proteins.

Ultimately, the Paleo diet aids in stabilizing blood sugar levels in the bloodstream, the burning of stored, excess fat, the reduction of allergies, infections, and inflammations, the strengthening of bones and teeth, the improvement of skin texture and complexion, the improvement of sleep patterns, and the maintenance of fantastic energy levels.

Vegan diet: In contrast to adherents of the Paleo diet, vegans refuse to consume anything of animal origin. In fact, they avoid anything with the word "animal" in it, including honey, silk, leather, wool, dairy products, cosmetics, detergents, etc. People may choose to become Vegan because they wish to maintain their health, are concerned about environmental degradation caused by animal agriculture, or are concerned about animal rights. Therefore, they concentrate solely on plant-based products. Vegans should not be confounded with vegetarians, who simply abstain from eating meat and eggs.

Cereal grains are essential to the vegan diet. This necessitates the inclusion of barley, wheat, cereals, bread, pasta, and rice. Five to seven servings of these grains per day, according to experts, are recommended for optimal health. Whole grains, which are typically fortified with other nutrients such as vitamin B 12, iron, and zinc, may be included in your daily diet if this is not feasible. Zinc is excellent for preventing cell and tissue degeneration and disease. Likewise, vitamin B 12 and iron are required for normal red blood cell production and the prevention of anemia.

Equally important for the correct functioning of the body are healthy fats. True, they should not be ingested in large quantities, but even the minimum daily intake is sufficient to maintain healthy body temperature regulation and organ health. Even your intellect will mature normally. Comparable to the Paleo diet, the Vegan diet emphasizes seeds, nuts, olive oil, Omega-3 fatty acids, canola oil, and nut butter, among other monounsaturated fat sources.

Vegans seek protein from nuts, soy, beans, and legumes because meat and seafood are considered forbidden. They obtain minerals such as iron from peas, dry legumes, soybeans, tofu, lentils, spinach, and fortified oatmeal. Oranges, tomatoes, asparagus, and strawberries are all excellent sources of vitamin C. Broccoli and dark-green foliage vegetables are excellent sources of calcium. Similar to the Paleo diet, an emphasis is placed on the consumption of organic vegetables and fruits.

Thus, the list of foodstuffs is virtually endless; these are merely a few examples of what may be consumed on a Vegan diet. Both the Paleo and Vegan diets emphasize balanced nutrition, which helps to maintain the health of organs and organ systems.

Begin Your Pegan Diet

Are you still uncertain about beginning this diet plan? You are uncertain about what you can ingest and what should be avoided or consumed in moderation. Let us assist you with these suggestions.

Vegetables and Fruits: To begin, ensure that the majority of the vegetables on your plate are dark or profound in color. These pigments indicate that you are consuming an abundance of natural phytonutrients. They will guarantee that your body remains free of disease. Therefore, incorporate vegetables into every meal. Yes, you need not limit yourself to dark-colored vegetables; if you must, embrace the entire plant kingdom. Some may be consumed fresh, while others require cooking. Regarding fruits, you may snack on them whenever you feel famished in between meals. Try to locate fruits grown organically; avoid hybrid varieties.

True, legumes are excellent sources of protein, minerals, and fiber; however, they can also cause digestive issues. They are also rich in carbohydrates, particularly the larger varieties. Consuming more than one cup of starch per day will result in the accumulation of excessive starch in the body. If you have prediabetes or diabetes, it is inevitable that your blood sugar levels will rise. Please limit your consumption of other legumes, such as peas, soy, lentils, etc., to a sensible level. As stated previously, they are difficult to assimilate.

Carbohydrates: It would be ideal to switch from white rice to brown rice, consuming no more than half a cup per meal. Other carbohydrate sources include white potatoes, parsnips, black rice (half a cup per meal), Winter Squash, Spaghetti Squash, Acorn Squash, plantains, sweet potatoes, coconut flour, almond flour, Quinoa (half a cup per meal), pumpkins, wild rice (half a cup per meal), coconut floor, Yam Noodles – Shirataki, etc. Ensure that your glycemic burden remains normal at all times. This means that a healthy balance of sugar and insulin should be present in the circulation. Otherwise, you put your heart, kidneys, liver, and other vital organs at risk for life-threatening diseases.

It may surprise you to learn that popular oils such as soybean oil, canola oil, sunflower oil, and maize oil are unhealthy for you. Omega-6 fatty acids are responsible for inflammation; soybean oil endures extensive processing. Coconut oil, sesame seed oil, avocado oil, olive oil, and Macadamia nut oil are preferable. Omega-3 lipids are beneficial to the heart and cholesterol levels. Yes, it is possible to discover Omega-3 fatty acids in meat from grass-fed or humanely raised animals. However, you should limit your consumption of these saturated lipids. Salmon, sardines, coconut milk, avocado, goat cheese, cashew butter, grass-fed butter, and almond butter are additional sources of healthful fats. You may include in your diet flax seeds, sesame seeds, hemp seeds, chia seeds, pumpkin seeds, walnuts, almonds, pistachios, and cashews.

Gluten: The type of wheat consumed by the majority of people today is referred to as "Franken wheat," which is quite distinct from the "Einkorn" or "Heirloom wheat" consumed in earlier centuries. Hybridization and crossbreeding have annihilated the original appearance and composition of the wheat that grew naturally in the past. Obviously, a great deal of virtue has also been destroyed. Gluten is abundant in whole cereals such as wheat, triticale, barley, and rye. Gluten is a glue-like protein. It has the ability to hold food together and preserve its shape. Where is wheat used the most? This ingredient can be found in baked products, cereals, breads, pasta, salad dressings, sauces, roux, and soups. Triticale is a comparatively contemporary grain used in pasta, cereals, and breads. Barley is present in vinegar, malt, soups, beer, and food coloring, whereas rye is present in rye bread and rye beer. This does cause confusion, doesn't it? However, take note of the following information in order to avoid gluten-containing foods as much as possible. Alternately, restrict their consumption to specific days of the week or month so they do not disrupt your blood sugar levels. Your body will produce antibodies that act against its own cells and tissues if you consume an excessive amount of gluten-containing whole grains.

True, you may have been a voracious meat eater up until now, but if you want to improve your health, you must drastically reduce your meat consumption. You must recognize that you are placing yourself at risk for obesity and diseases associated with obesity. You could consider it as a side dish as opposed to the main course. This indicates that it should constitute approximately 25% of your supper, along with 75% of black rice, sweet potatoes, winter squash, etc. It would be beneficial to choose beef from grass-fed livestock or cattle raised sustainably. You will be able to store Omega-3 fatty acids, vitamin A, vitamin D, cholesterol-free stearic acid, and antioxidants. As for fish, sardines, wild salmon, etc. have lower mercury levels and higher amounts of healthy fatty acids; you will be secure if you consume these.

Sugar: It would be best to treat it as an occasional indulgence as soon as you commence your vegan diet. Stop adding excessive quantities of sugar to every recipe, oversweetening your coffee and tea, consuming sugary condiments, and gorging on sugary cereals, for instance. It does not matter what form sugar takes; it is never wholesome. Instead, use coconut sugar, organic honey, or raw maple syrup in sensible quantities as substitutes. Since they are minimally processed, they are healthier for you.

According to researchers, dairy products derived from bovines are liable for a number of obesity-related illnesses. Furthermore, they may increase the risk of osteoporosis. You may occasionally attempt goat and sheep-derived organic products as an alternative. Alternatively, you could substitute soymilk or coconut milk for milk in your morning cereal. There are numerous diet-friendly milk products available; just consult with an expert.

Processed foods: Every type of nutritional program on the planet recommends avoiding or limiting the consumption of extensively processed foods at all costs. Yet, in an effort to meet stringent deadlines and adhere to predetermined schedules, you ensure that tins and cans from supermarket and department store shelves easily enter your home. Your body does not require artificial preservatives, edible compounds, additives, artificial sweeteners, artificial colors, or MSG. It also does not require excess fat. If you continue your current behaviors, you will load your body with toxic substances, which will increase the size of your stomach, abdomen, buttocks, upper limbs, and lower limbs.

What To Consume & What To Avoid

With all of this information about how your diet affects your short- and long-term health, you're presumably wondering what foods you can consume. To create a diet that will maximize your health and longevity and prevent serious diseases, you must first discover what foods you can consume.

Although the vegan diet restricts many foods, it is not as restrictive as you may believe. There are always instances when certain foods are acceptable, and a fear of eliminating foods will make it more difficult to do so. Simply make an effort to live a 90% vegan lifestyle and always do what is best for your body.

The pegan diet permits the majority of fruits and vegetables, gluten-free grains, proteins from sustainable sources, and omega-3-rich nuts and seeds. These dietary groups were selected by Dr. Hyman for very specific reasons.

Foods to Enjoy

The pegan diet emphasizes eating delicious fruits and vegetables, meat, nuts, seeds, eggs, and fish. Unlike many other diets, the primary focus of the pegan diet is on eating nutrient-rich, whole foods and eliminating foods that cause us to bloat, spike our blood sugar, and drain us of energy. Let's talk about the categories of foods that you will grow to appreciate even more.

Fruits and Vegetables

Eating organic, non-starchy vegetables is essential for complete veganism. Nature provides us with an abundance of vegetables and fruits to appreciate. These plants are natural remedies for a variety of diseases and health issues. Fruits and vegetables are also delicious.

Once you eradicate many products with added sugar, you will discover that many fruits and vegetables are naturally quite sweet. Nature provides us with natural glucose, which will satisfy most sweet desires. The amount of sugar added to candies, cakes, and processed delicacies is frequently excessive. After removing these foods from your diet, you will gradually adjust to the delicate flavor of fruits.

Vegetables such as organic artichokes, asparagus, avocado, bean sprouts, Brussels sprouts, broccoli, cabbage, cauliflower, celery, cucumber, eggplant, garlic, ginger, and leafy greens should be consumed on the vegan diet. As much as possible, consume peppers, onions, mushrooms, radicchio, rutabaga, seaweed, scallions, and squash. Find methods to incorporate tomatoes, turnips, and zucchini, along with sweet potatoes, yams, and pumpkin.

As for fruit, consume organic blackberries, cranberries, kiwi, blueberries, lemons, limes, and raspberries that are low in glycemic index. Avoid using high-glycemic fruit beverages to meet your daily fruit requirement.

Nuts & Seeds

Nuts and seeds play an essential role in the pegan diet in protecting us from harmful diseases and balancing our blood sugar. Fortunately, nuts and seeds are versatile and can be incorporated into a variety of delectable dishes. Add seeds and nuts to all of your meals, from nutbars to salad toppings and even dessert.

The diet of ancient humans is largely responsible for the importance of nuts and seeds. This is the 'paleo' component of being pegan. Our paleolithic ancestors consumed omega-6 and omega-3 fatty acids in a 1:1 ratio. When in balance, these acids are anti-inflammatory and aid in blood coagulation. However, these effects are reversed when our diet contains a greater ratio of omega-6 to omega-3. A "junk-food and fast-food diet" has a ratio of 20 to 1, indicating an elevated level of inflammation in the body.

Nuts and seeds contain a healthy balance of omega-3 and omega-6 fatty acids, making them exceptionally beneficial for the body. In addition, they are abundant in fiber, vitamins, protein, carbohydrates, minerals, and antioxidants. Walnuts, hemp seeds, flaxseeds, and chia seeds contain the highest levels of omega-3 fatty acids and nutrients derived from plants.

The pegan diet permits the consumption of nuts such as almonds, Brazil nuts, cashews, hazelnuts, macadamia nuts, pecans, pine nuts, pistachios, walnuts, and organic cacao. Regarding seeds, you should consume chia, flax, hemp, pumpkin, sesame, and sunflower.

Grains

Gluten-free whole carbohydrates are excellent for the body. Grains contain protein, fiber, and minerals that support the immune system. On the vegan diet, you are encouraged to consume approximately 1/2 cup of the following whole grains daily: quinoa, black rice, brown rice, red rice, wild rice, teff, amaranth, and buckwheat. These are outstanding side dishes or primary courses.

On the vegan diet, oatmeal and gluten-free grains are also permitted. About a half-cup is the maximum serving size for these foods. Oatmeal contains a specific type of fiber that keeps you feeling full for an extended period of time throughout the day. This means spending less time desiring unhealthy foods and more time concentrating on what's important.

Beans

Beans are frequently the subject of debate among dietitians, but in actuality, beans possess many positive qualities that are essential to our diet. By selecting the correct beans to consume, you can anticipate numerous health benefits.

The initial step in selecting the proper beans is to select well-prepared beans. Avoid canned beans because certain varieties of cans contain the hormone disruptor bisphenol A (BPA). Make an effort to locate BPA-free canned legumes. The most effective method for preparing legumes is to soak them in salted water overnight. You might consider planning your meals for the week to make this task more manageable.

After selecting beans that have been properly prepared, choose legumes that will provide fiber and protein without causing a blood sugar spike. Lupini beans, green beans, lentils, miso, tempeh, chickpeas, black beans, snap peas, and snow peas are delicious.

Meats and Fish

Dr. Hyman recommends consuming a maximum of 4-6 ounces of animal protein twice per day. It is essential to consume pasture-raised, antibiotic- and hormone-free animal protein. Purchase animal products that are humanely and ethically raised.

Indulge in organic meats such as turkey, duck, pheasant, lamb, beef, bison, venison, deer, and elk. Shrimp, wild salmon, clams, cod, crab, flounder, herring, mussels, sardines, scallops, and trout are delectable seafood options.

On a pegan diet, cow's milk should be limited. In moderation, you may consume grass-fed butter, ghee, goat and sheep yogurt, and cheese.

The key to selecting meat is ensuring that it comes from a source that prioritizes your health and the health of the animals. Additionally, meat production and exploitation have significant effects on the environment. Limiting our meat consumption to lean meats and seafood is beneficial for our bodies, the environment, and our well-being.

Water It is essential to replenish your body's water supply. Keep yourself hydrated throughout the day for optimal results. Fresh, purified water will aid in body detoxification, digestion improvement, and vitality maximization.

Additionally, you may consume herbal tea, seltzer, mineral water, or green beverages throughout the day. As long as your body responds healthily to caffeine, consuming coffee or caffeine is acceptable. For instance, palpitations or digestive issues caused by coffee are your body's way of communicating that it doesn't like it or that you've consumed too much.

Regarding alcohol, Dr. Hyman recommends one glass of wine per week or three cocktails per week. Like everything else on the vegan diet, alcohol can be consumed in moderation.

Sugar

Sugar is ubiquitous in grocery stores, even in products that are not typically associated with being sugary, such as bacon and white bread. These substances raise blood sugar levels, resulting in insulin resistance. This is something you should avoid, especially because it causes type 2 diabetes and other serious health problems.

Then, does sugar have a role in the vegan diet? The answer is affirmative, in moderation. There are times in everyone's life when a delicious treat is a part of the celebration and the recollections.

However, there is a distinction between occasionally savoring sugar and making it a daily habit. On the pegan diet, sucrose can be consumed occasionally. If you desire to improve your health, however, it cannot become a daily routine. The overwhelming majority of your diet should be composed of whole, natural foods.

Additionally, consuming sugar does not necessitate purchasing commercially-produced foods. Instead of purchasing pre-made sugary foods, the dessert segment of this book can be used to create your own sweet treats. Some of these recipes utilize the natural sugar produce and require no additional ingredients.

If your recipe calls for sugar, choose your sugar carefully. Stevia, monk fruit, maple syrup, honey, coconut sugar, and date sugar are acceptable in small quantities. These chemical compounds are significantly more beneficial to the body than refined cane sugar.

Scarce Foods

While everything can be enjoyed in moderation, there are certain nutrients that your body does not require. By removing these foods from your diet, you eliminate a variety of health problems and afflictions. You are improving your health in a number of ways, from reducing your risk of heart disease to eradicating the possibility of developing type 2 diabetes.

Here is a list of ingredients that are not permitted on a vegan diet, as well as an explanation of why and how to avoid them. This list includes non-whole foods, gluten, conventional dairy, refined oils and sugars. These foods should be replaced with nutrient-dense, unadulterated whole foods that lack additives, preservatives, and lengthy chemical names.

Items that are not Whole

The pegan diet prioritizes whole, nutrient-dense foods. Please avoid processed and artificial foods that have been altered from their natural state. This includes flour and refined wheat products. Avoid processed wheat foods, potato snacks, and other artificial foods designed to induce addiction.

To combat the desire to consume processed foods, maintain a constant supply of low-glycemic fruits and non-starchy vegetables. Use the snack concoctions described in 8 to satisfy your hunger.

Finished Oils

Grass-fed ghee, avocado oil, or organic extra virgin coconut oil, almond oil, flax oil, hemp oil, macadamia oil, and extra virgin olive oil should be the only oils and condiments used.

The gut microbiome is a delicate ecosystem of microorganisms that consume whatever you consume. An dysfunctional microbiome can result in a variety of diseases. Refined vegetable oils nourish pathogenic microbes and cause intestinal permeability and inflammation. This can result in illness and disease.

These substances are extremely harmful to the body. Check the oils contained in every product you purchase, including food served in restaurants and cafes. Put excellent oils in your pantry and get rid of the ones that will cause you more trouble in the long run.

Too Much Sugar & Starch

Sugar and starch are ubiquitous in fast food and junk cuisine. From hamburger buns to fries to packaged bread, these two constituents are ubiquitous in processed foods. Consuming whole foods and avoiding starchy vegetables will enable you to avoid their negative effects.

Sugar is a highly addictive ingredient that is added in large proportions to a variety of processed foods. However, sugar is not an essential nutrient for the human organism. It is a wholly unnecessary ingredient that disrupts the body's chemistry when consumed in excess.

When consumed, starch and sugar both produce a chain reaction in the body. It causes an immediate insulin rise, resulting in a brief surge of energy. This results in the development of insulin resistance in the organism. The greater your consumption of carbohydrates and sugar, the higher your insulin levels will be.

With increased insulin levels and insulin resistance, the body resorts to 1) fat storage and 2) inflammation. An inundation of sugar and starch is also detrimental to the microbiome. Therefore, it begins to produce chemicals that induce a rapid decline in mood.

You may question if you should completely eliminate sugar from your diet in light of these negative effects. The pegan diet excludes foods that are detrimental to health, but sugar and carbohydrate can be consumed in moderation. Selecting carbohydrate vegetables and natural sugars are the healthiest alternatives for occasional consumption.

Consider sugar to be a recreational substance. It provides no nutritional value to the body, so its sole function is entertainment. Instead of adding sugar to everything you eat, save the sweetener for something genuinely delectable and use maple syrup or honey instead.

Meat, milk products, and animal protein

There is considerable debate regarding whether or not animal protein is healthy. Our earliest ancestors relied on animal protein from hunting animals and consumed a variety of vegetation, seeds, and nuts. Reducing animal protein consumption is generally a good idea for the reasons stated earlier.

Limit your consumption of lunch meat, hot dogs, and prosciutto, as well as meats that are unethically sourced and overly processed. Many of these meats contain cancer-causing compounds, hormones, and antibiotics that have negative effects on human health.

Cow's milk causes inflammation in the digestive system, which leads to subsequent digestive issues. Most people lack the enzymes required to break down lactose, causing inflammation throughout the body. Milk is also a part of the unethical cycle of livestock production, which is a practice that none of us should support.

There are also corrupt practices associated with fish, such as ocean pollution and disruption of food chains. In addition to antibiotics and dietary supplements, farmed fish are also fed substances that we subsequently digest. The ideal option is to consume wild-caught fish that is rich in omega-3 and omega-6 fatty acids.

Strategies for Reducing Food Intake

Eliminating food from our diet may appear unfeasible. This is particularly true when the food group is consumed frequently. Here are six strategies for eliminating food groups from your diet that will help you get over the initial hurdle of a new eating regimen.

If possible, remove all non-vegan foods from your larder and refrigerator. When your stomach is rumbling, seeing a bag of potato crisps does not make the transition to veganism easier. When goods are within arms' reach, it is simple to obtain them. By removing all unhealthy food and processed foods from your pantry, the transition to a vegan diet will be ten times simpler.

Display fruits and vegetables more aesthetically. Observe how candy is always the first item that catches your eye in the checkout lane of a grocery store. Children will implore their parents for Skittles, M&Ms, or chocolate, to name a few, if the candies are placed at eye level in grocery stores. Utilize this psychological tip in the kitchen. Store fruits in acrylic glass containers and position them in a visible location in the refrigerator. Remove the flimsy plastic sacks that conceal the colorful skin of vegetables and display them in their natural state for all to see.

Additionally, prepare fruits, vegetables, nuts, and seeds for sustenance in advance. Most people won't feel like chopping a bell pepper at the moment, but chopping the crunchy and colorful peppers beforehand makes them a simple snack. The same holds true for other pagan foods, such as fruit and seeds. Make healthful eating simple in your home.

Prepare your dishes in advance to eliminate mealtime decisions. By preparing meals at the start of the week, you reduce tension and decision-making. Additionally, worrying about what you're going to cook can cause you to make unhealthy but convenient decisions.

According to Dr. Hyman, 90% of the time, you should be pegan. You need not fear never again consuming cake or missing out on baseball hotdogs. As long as you strive to consume pegan the majority of the time, you are doing well. Your health, digestion, and longevity are improving.

Plan tasty, simple recipes that inspire you. This compendium contains numerous recipes that can be prepared by anyone. Be inventive in the kitchen and learn to cook at home to save money on dining out.

Please exercise extreme patience with yourself. Perhaps you are new to the vegan or paleo diet. If this is the case, it is recommended to implement changes gradually. There are numerous foods that you can and cannot consume, and it can be intimidating to discover these new lists. Keep in mind that your body is a machine that can be resistant to abrupt change. Try incorporating progressively more fruits and vegetables and decreasing your consumption of animal products.

Some Pegan Diet Rules

mitigating irritation. To comprehend the rules for adhering to a Pegan diet, the following must be considered:

1. Select Seasonal Fruits and Vegetables

Seventy-five percent of your plate should be comprised of verdant greens for a Pegan diet. In reality, they should be a significant part of your daily diet. They contain minerals and nutrients that keep you healthy and protect you from illness.

For a more active, healthy, normal, and balanced lifestyle, the majority of people would benefit from consuming more vegetables and organic foods. Vegetables and natural products contain a variety of minerals and nutrients that are beneficial to your health, such as folic acid, phosphorus, zinc, magnesium, as well as vitamins E, C, A (beta-carotene), etc.

Similarly, fruits and vegetables are low in sugar, sodium, and fat. They are important sources of dietary filaments and low in calories. You will want to maintain a healthy weight and reduce your waist circumference with the aid of soil-based products. Additionally, you will reduce your blood pressure and cholesterol levels.

Fruits and vegetables contain potent phytochemicals that help protect your overall health. Phytochemicals are ordinarily associated with hue; consequently, vegetables and natural products of various hues, including white, blue-purple, red, yellow-orange, and green, contain their own blend of vitamins and phytochemicals that work together to promote health. For instance, white vegetables such as cauliflower contain sulforaphane, which may protect against certain types of cancer; whereas, green vegetables such as kale and spinach contain zeaxanthin and lutein, which protect against age-related medical conditions such as eye diseases.

We will discuss the Rainbow diet in greater detail later in this section.

To increase supplement consumption, it is essential to ingest a variety of soil-based products. You can try purchasing leafy foods according to the seasons; this is nature's way of ensuring that your body receives a healthy combination of plant chemicals and supplements. Alternatively, you may decide to purchase various agricultural products and experiment with new recipes.

2. Quality Is Essential

Remembered foods for a Pegan diet are referred to as authentic food sources; these food varieties are rich in nutrients, free of chemical additives, and generally natural. In general, these are the types of dietary sources that the earliest human populations consumed. Tragically, the twentieth century witnessed an explosion in the popularity of processed and ready-to-eat foods.

While processed foods are advantageous and convenient, they are also harmful to the human body. Indeed, consuming authentic, high-quality food sources is one of the most important things you can do for your body to maintain a high-quality life and excellent health. The types of foods you consume will determine your overall health.

For the condition of any diet, the nature of the food varieties and ingredients is essential. The essence of the food sources for a vegan diet should essentially be phenomenal. A typical Pegan dish must contain two to three cups of fresh produce, including a variety of non-boring greens and other vegetables. To achieve the greatest nutrient density, it is also recommended to combine gorgeous vegetables and organic products. Due to the emphasis on quality in a Pegan diet, it is recommended to choose organic and privately grown foods whenever possible.

A Pegan diet also consists of several animal-based foods. Regardless, these dishes are intended to be served alongside the plant-based main courses.

The eggs, poultry, and red meat should be reared humanely or on grass. The fish should be captured in the wild and contain less mercury.

Omega-3 unsaturated lipids are also a component of a Pegan diet; omega-3 fat sources are renowned for their potent anti-inflammatory properties. These dietary types typically include fish, which must be wild-caught fatty fish such as herring, mackerel, anchovies, sardines, and salmon.

3. You should consume 75% of your calories from plant foods.

A Pegan diet is a blend of a paleo diet and a veggie lover diet. The paleo diet consists of whole food sources that our ancestors hunted and gathered, such as vegetables, organic products, and occasionally meat. However, the vegetarian diet entails consuming only plant-based items.

A Pegan diet is, by definition, one that consists of 75% plant-based dietary sources and 25% animal-based protein. These food sources should be complete and economically produced while minimizing their environmental impact.

Although there have been no conclusive studies demonstrating the health benefits of a Pegan diet, experts are accumulating evidence that the semi-vegetarian diet is beneficial to health. Since a plant-based diet focuses on vegetables and fruits that are low in starch and high in fiber, a Pegan diet is thought to be the finest type of diet available today. A plant-based diet has also been shown to reduce bad cholesterol levels in the body and promote weight loss.

Vegetables and organic products are the most nutrient-dense and healthiest food types available today; they contain the highest levels of minerals and nutrients that can aid in disease prevention and reduce inflammation and oxidative stress.

Despite this, there are certain types of plant-based food sources that you should avoid. For instance, white bread and rice are also examples of plant-based foods. However, they are intensively processed, which renders them devoid of body-nourishing nutrients and high in glycemic index. Thus, this can result in increased appetite (which leads to overeating) and elevated glucose levels.

The remaining 25% of the diet consists of animal-based proteins. Regardless, portions should be small; consider all meat dishes to be side dishes. The sources of flesh should be field-raised and grass-fed. Regarding fish, it should come from the wild and contain as little mercury as possible.

Eat the Spectrum

For the healthiest diet, experts recommend consuming all the colors of the rainbow. As mentioned previously, this suggests that you consume vibrant vegetables and organic foods. These have numerous positive effects on the organism.

Plants contain a variety of pigments, also known as phytonutrients. These phytonutrients give them a wide variety of hues. Different-hued vegetables and natural products are frequently associated with particular health benefits and supplements. While consuming a large amount of verdant foods is beneficial, it is also important to focus on consuming a variety of colored vegetables in order to increase your intake of various vitamins and minerals for the benefit of your overall health.

While phytonutrients have numerous advantages, it is not simple to conduct randomized controlled trials; as a result, specialists have organized their research according to the admissions and disease risk of the population. According to these studies, it has been determined that consuming colorful vegetables and natural products has numerous benefits and almost no drawbacks. You will provide your body with an assortment of phytochemicals, minerals, and vitamins by incorporating shading into your Pegan diet.

Anti-inflammatory

In the past couple of years, the phrases 'without gluten' and 'lactose-free' have appeared everywhere. Many individuals who are no longer gluten-dependent have figured out how to manage persistent infections, food intolerances, and stress. Dairy and gluten are common allergens that can cause numerous health problems in humans.

Gluten is a type of prolamin protein commonly found in cereals such as rye, grain, and wheat. Gluten is frequently referred to as "magic" that binds prepared foods due to its elasticity.

There are numerous ways in which gluten can irritate the body. This is due to the fact that it contains indisputable amounts of enemies of supplements, which are plant-based proteins.

These supplement foes are harmful to the body because they inhibit the normal digestion and absorption of food in the stomach, causing inflammation.

Additionally, gluten consumption induces zonulin production in the body. Zonulin is a type of protein in the body that regulates the opening and closing of stomach mucosal junctions. Our stomach is particularly permeable, allowing beneficial substances to enter the circulatory system while storing harmful substances for expulsion. When zonulin is removed, the stomach's permeability will decrease and the intersections will remain open.

Milk from sheep, goats, cows, and even camels is referred to as dairy. In addition to margarine, cheddar, kefir, yogurt, and milk, dairy is present in a variety of other products. Dairy is categorized as an allergenic substance that is difficult to digest, which causes inflammation.

For instance, lactose intolerance is a condition caused by dairy. Lactose is a sugar found in milk; for the body to metabolize lactose, it must produce the enzyme lactase. This protein is produced in the body during adolescence, but we lose the ability to produce it as we age. This is an extremely common condition, as over 65 percent of adults worldwide are lactose intolerant.

Casein, a protein found in dairy products, can cause problems with secure framework function and assimilation, particularly A1 casein. If you believe lactose and A1 casein are causing stomach-related issues, you can seek out alternative dairy options. Goat's milk contains less lactose than cow's milk, for example.

6. Say No to Vegetable Oils

Vegetable oils are detrimental to your health and the environment, a fact that is not widely known. Vegetable oils consist of oils extracted from seeds such as nut, safflower, sunflower, maize, soybean, and rapeseed (canola oil). Unlike olive oil and coconut oil, which are extracted by pressing, these vegetable oils are extracted in an unnatural manner.

In addition to the persistent myths about cholesterol and saturated fats, these oils are frequently promoted as healthy because they contain omega-3 unsaturated fats and monounsaturated fats. These false health claims will be a frequent focus of future developments. Nonetheless, this does not explain the overall picture.

Vegetable oils contain high concentrations of polyunsaturated fatty acids (PUFAs), whereas the human body is composed of 97% monounsaturated and saturated lipids. The fat is necessary for hormone production and cell repair. PUFAs, on the other hand, are extremely unstable and rapidly oxidize. This can then result in cell mutation and inflammation. The oxidation has also been associated with other heart-related diseases.

We are all aware that omega-3 fatty acids are extremely beneficial. However, the ratio of omega-3 to omega-6 fatty acids is essential for optimal health.

Many omega-6 fatty acids are present in vegetable oils. These acids are rapidly oxidized. On the other hand, it has been shown that omega-3 fatty acids protect against cancer and reduce inflammation. Unbalanced levels of both types of acids have been associated with various malignancies and other health issues.

In addition to the unnatural levels of omega-6 fatty acids and polyunsaturated lipids, these vegetable oils also contain chemicals, pesticides, and processing additives. Some also contain the natural antioxidants BHT and BHA, which prevent the food from spoiling rapidly. However, research has shown that they also produce cancer-causing compounds in the body. Additionally, vegetable oil is associated with kidney and liver injury, behavioral issues, infertility, and immune system problems.

7. Avoid sugar and consume fruits sparingly.

Almost all products, from peanut butter to marinara sauce, contain added sugar. The majority of people eat processed foods for snacks and supper. However, these products also contain added sugar, which contributes significantly to their calorie content.

According to dietary guidelines, you should consume no more than 10% of your daily calories from added sugar. It has been determined that excessive sugar consumption is the leading cause of obesity and can also contribute to a variety of chronic diseases, such as Type 2 diabetes.

The rates of obesity are higher than ever before, and sugar-sweetened beverages are a major contributor. Fructose is a basic sugar found in sugar-sweetened beverages such as sweet tea, juice, and soda. When fructose is consumed, appetite increases. Additionally, fructose increases resistance to leptin, a hormone that regulates appetite and signals the body to cease eating.

In brief, sugary beverages do not satisfy hunger, and you end up consuming excessive calories from liquids, leading to weight gain. According to research, those who consume sweetened beverages are heavier than those who do not.

A diet elevated in sugar can also increase the risk of developing cardiovascular disease. High-sugar diets have been linked to inflammation, obesity, and elevated blood pressure, all of which are risk factors for a variety of cardiac conditions.

Increased sugar intake has also been associated with acne. Foods with a high glycemic index, such as processed sugary delights, raise blood sugar levels more rapidly than foods with a low GMI. These foods will cause insulin and blood sugar levels to rise, resulting in increased inflammation, oil production, and androgen secretion, all of which contribute to acne. In addition, population studies have revealed that rural areas of the globe that consume unprocessed foods have virtually no acne, compared to high-income areas and cities.

8. Avoid Gluten Grains

As stated previously, gluten is a naturally occurring protein present in cereals such as rye, barley, and wheat. This substance has a stretchy aspect and is responsible for holding the food together. Triticale, einkorn, Khorasan wheat, graham, farro, farina, semolina, emmer, durum, spelt, and wheat berries are additional grains that contain gluten. Although oats are naturally gluten-free, cross-contamination occurs during processing with the grains enumerated previously. Additionally, modified food starch and soy sauce are less apparent sources of gluten.

The downside of gluten is that it can induce side effects in some individuals. When the immune system recognizes gluten as a pathogen, it will launch an attack against it. If you are gluten-sensitive and accidentally consume gluten, you will experience inflammation. Mild side effects include diarrhea, alternating constipation, bloating, and fatigue, while severe side effects include intestinal injury, malnutrition, and unintended weight loss.

An estimated one in 113 Americans has celiac disease, and it has been determined that those with celiac disease have a higher risk of anemia and osteoporosis. This results in additional health issues, including nerve disorders, infertility, and even cancer.

The positive news is that the damage can be reversed by removing gluten from one's diet. A gluten-free diet is frequently the solution for celiac disease. However, adhering to a gluten-free diet is not simple; you may need the assistance of a registered dietitian to determine which foods contain gluten and to find gluten-free substitutes for other essential nutrients.

In brief, a gluten-free diet is a diet that prohibits the consumption of gluten-containing foods. However, the majority of gluten-containing whole grains also contain iron, magnesium, and vitamins. Therefore, it is essential that you replenish these nutrients. For example, you can consider poultry, eggs, fish, nuts, and whole fruits and vegetables as inherently gluten-free foods.

9. Include Nutritious Fats

The majority of individuals are unable to comprehend why monounsaturated and polyunsaturated fats are beneficial to the body and why trans fats are harmful. In fact, we have been attempting to eliminate lipids from your diets whenever possible by recommending low-fat meals. However, this change does not enhance our health because healthy fats are reduced alongside unhealthy fats.

While some lipids are detrimental to the human body, others are essential. Fats are one of the most essential energy sources for the human organism. It will aid in mineral and vitamin absorption. Additionally, fats contribute to the formation of sheaths surrounding nerves and cell membranes. Additionally, fats are beneficial for inflammation, muscle movement, and blood coagulation. Consequently, certain fats are beneficial to the body in the long term.

All lipids, whether healthy or unhealthy, share a similar chemical structure. It is composed of a chain of carbon atoms and hydrogen atoms. The only distinction between these fats is the number, size, and configuration of the hydrogen and carbon atoms, respectively.

Before discussing the excellent and healthy fats, let's examine the unhealthy fats. Trans fat is the most dangerous form of fat. This fat is produced when hydrogenation is used to transform healthful oils into solids to prevent rancidity. This form of fat has no health benefits and is also unsafe for consumption. In fact, trans fat has been prohibited in countries such as the United States.

In contrast, polyunsaturated and monounsaturated lipids are healthy fats found primarily in fish, seeds, nuts, and vegetables. At room temperature, this form of fat remains liquid.

When you submerge your bread into olive oil, you consume monounsaturated fat. This fat contains a solitary carbon-to-carbon double bond, resulting in two fewer hydrogen atoms. Monounsaturated lipids remain liquid at room temperature for this reason. Sunflower oils, almonds, avocados, peanut oil, and olive oil are excellent sources of monounsaturated fats.

Consume Clean Meat, Poultry, and Whole Eggs

As previously stated, meat and poultry are excellent sources of protein for a Pegan diet. In addition, they contain many essential nutrients, such as essential fatty acids, vitamins, zinc, iron, and iodine. As a result, it is always advisable to include poultry, meat, and eggs in a Pegan diet. To avoid consuming saturated fat and salt, however, it is recommended that you adhere to lean and unprocessed cuts.

Clean eating is an amorphous concept, signifying that there are no caloric or dietary restrictions. Avoiding packaged and processed foods that are high in artificial ingredients, sodium, and sugar appears to be the common denominator of clean eating when it comes to whole eggs, meat, and poultry. Thus, you choose whole or natural animal-based goods over processed ones.

Eggs, poultry, and meat should be purchased fresh, unseasoned, and free of artificial ingredients. These foods are nutritionally dense, high in protein, and minimal in fat by design.

After ensuring that you have purchased clean meat, cooking will eliminate all bacteria and other microorganisms. In addition to being nutritious, it will safeguard you and your family against food poisoning.

Some poultry and meat products must be cooked thoroughly; this means that the juices should flow clear and there should be no pink or red meat when you cut into them. The following are examples of meats and poultry that must be cooked thoroughly:

Rolled flesh products

Kebabs

Sausages and rissoles

organ meats (including liver)

Pork

All varieties of poultry and game,
including duck, goose, turkey, and fowl

However, there are also meats that can
be eaten when they are rare or brown in
the center. These are just a few:

roasted meats

Cutlets

Steaks

Depending on the quality and size of the flesh cut, cooking will be clean. Consequently, you should focus more on monitoring the temperature than the preparation time.

Preparing To Go Pegan

Today, it is common for individuals to begin a Pegan diet; it is the newest diet trend. Can you consume meat? Yes, but you should not exaggerate.

What about manufactured substances? You can only consume a few. This diet consists primarily of whole foods, so you will consume fresh vegetables and fruits.

The Pegan diet is a combination of the vegan and paleo diets based on the theory that whole foods promote optimal health by reducing inflammation and balancing blood sugar.

Combining vegan and paleo diets may appear contradictory or strange at first sight. However, rest assured that this is not the case. You should view it as a compromise that combines the finest aspects of both diets.

Meal planning is fundamentally straightforward. As stated previously,

Pegan diet recipes include modest quantities of high-quality animal-based proteins, an abundance of healthy fat, and fruits and vegetables. In addition, you must avoid legumes (peanuts, lentils, peas, and beans), cereals, and dairy products.

Vegan and paleo diets both adhere to the following program tenets:

Fats from olive oil, seeds, almonds, avocados, and omega-3 fatty acids are of superior quality.

Consider organic, hormone- and antibiotic-free, and non-GMO foods as pesticide-free.

Absolutely no chemicals: No MSG, artificial colors, flavors, or additives.

Look for vegetables and fruits with intense and vibrant hues; the greater the variety, the better.

Low in refined carbohydrates, flour, and sugar

If you choose to follow the Pegan regimen, you will:

Consume saccharine products sparingly; you can enjoy them on occasion.

Avoid legumes, cereals, and dairy

Consume an abundance of seeds and almonds because their high protein content reduces the risk of diabetes and cardiovascular disease.

Vegetables should comprise approximately 75% of your daily diet.

Consume the proper lipids, such as omega-3, seeds, olive oil, nuts, and avocados; avoid soy and vegetable oils.

Consume foods with a low glycemic load; instead, seek out more fats and proteins in foods such as sardines, olive oil, seeds, and almonds.

Controversy

Since 2014, Pegan recipes and diet have risen dramatically in popularity. In 2021, Pinterest searches for 'consuming Pegan' increased by 337%. However, this regimen has also generated some controversy.

For instance, experts have suggested that the general parameters of this diet are merely the combination of two opposing diet philosophies. In reality, they believe that the majority of Pegan diet restrictions are time-consuming, expensive, and unnecessary.

According to these nutritional and dietary authorities, limiting legumes could be problematic, for instance. According to studies, legumes are low in cholesterol, high in fiber, and a rich source of protein, making them an essential component of the widely popular Mediterranean diet. In addition, legumes have been associated with a variety of health benefits, such as the prevention of cardiovascular disease, cancer, and others.

Optimistic Reports

While there have been some debates about the Pegan diet, there have also been numerous positive responses. The majority of experts concur with Dr. Hyman that animal-based products should be ingested as condiments and not as the main course. Additionally, scientists adore the notion of increasing vegetable, fruit, and seafood consumption.

Others have concurred that there are numerous aspects of a Pegan diet, such as the emphasis on omega-3 fatty acids, fruits, and vegetables, and adequate protein. The conclusion is that a Pegan diet may be beneficial to your health. Nevertheless, there are certain restrictions that you must observe. If you can do so, the Pegan diet will begin to have a beneficial effect on your body.

One-Skillet Kale And Avocado

Ingredients

- 1 avocado, sliced

- 4 large whole eggs

- Salt and pepper as needed

- 2 tablespoons olive oil, divided

- 2 cups mushrooms, sliced

- 5 ounces fresh kale, stemmed and sliced into ribbons

Directions

1.   Take a large skillet and place it over medium heat

2.   Add a tablespoon of olive oil

3.   Add mushrooms to the pan and Saute for 1-5 minutes

4.   Take a medium bowl and massage kale with the remaining 1 tablespoon olive oil

5.   Add kale to skillet and place them on top of mushrooms

6.   Place slices of avocado on top of the kale

7.   Create 1-5 wells for eggs and crack each egg onto each hold

8.   Season eggs with salt and pepper

9.   Cover skillet and cook for 10-15 minutes

10. Serve hot!

Soup With Roasted Butternut Squash

Ingredients:

- ½ cup diced yellow onion
- 1 medium green apple, cored and chopped
- 3 cups low-sodium chicken or vegetable broth
- ½ teaspoon ground cumin
- 1 (5 lbs.) butternut squash, peeled, seeded and chopped
- 2 to 3 tablespoons olive oil
- 1 teaspoon ground cinnamon
- Salt to taste
- 2 tablespoons coconut oil
- 1 cup chopped carrots

Instructions:

1. Preheat the oven to 450°F.

2. Toss the butternut squash with the olive oil, cinnamon and salt.

3. Spread the squash on a baking sheet and roast for 35 to 40 minutes, stirring once.

4. Heat the coconut oil in a stockpot over medium heat.

5. Stir in the roasted butternut squash along with the carrots, apple, and onion.

6. Add the chicken broth and cumin then season with salt to taste.

7. Bring the mixture to boil and then reduce heat and simmer for 35 to 40 minutes, covered.

8. Remove from heat and puree the soup using an immersion blender. Serve hot.

Toasted Coconut Cha Dessert

Ingredients

- 2 pinch sea salt

- ¼ cup chia seeds

- ½ cup unsweetened shredded coconut

- 4 cups cubed tropical fruit (mango, pineapple, etc.)

- 2 cup unsweetened plain almond milk

- 2 cup coconut milk

- 2 teaspoon lime juice

- 4 tablespoons maple syrup

- 2 teaspoon vanilla extract

- ½ cup chia seeds

Instructions

1. First, whisk together the coconut milk, maple syrup, lime juice, vanilla extract, and sea salt.
2. Next, add the chia seeds and whisk for an additional 1-5 minutes.
3. Then, rest at room temperature for about 35 to 40 minutes, whisking occasionally.
4. Second , refrigerate the pudding for at least three hours.

5. However, chilling it overnight works best.

6. Third, add the coconut to a large non-stick skillet and toast over medium heat for about 1-5 minutes until light brown.

7. Fourth, stir the pudding and add to single-serving sized bowls,

8. Then, top with the cubed tropical fruit and toasted coconut. Serve immediately.

Lime Dressed Avocado And Coriander Salad

- 1 small green chilli pepper
- salt
- white pepper
- 2 limes
- 3 avocados
- ½ fret coriander

1. Wash the limes in hot water, pat dry, rub a small amount of peel off, and squeeze the limes.
2. Remove the stones from the avocados and cut them in half.
3. Cut the pulp into wedges and dice it after peeling off the peel.
4. Combine the avocado cubes and lime juice in a mixing bowl.
5. Coriander should be washed, shaken dry, and finely chopped before being mixed with the avocado cubes.

6. Remove the stone and the white inner skin from the chili pepper, then cut the pulp into fine cubes.
7. Toss the salad with the chili cubes. Season with salt and pepper to taste, then steep for 55 to 60 minutes.
8. Allow to cool slightly before serving.

www.ingramcontent.com/pod-product-compliance
Lightning Source LLC
Chambersburg PA
CBHW060503030426
42337CB00015B/1713